#dietGOALS

For general information on our other products and services or to obtain technical support, please contact our Customer Care Department within the United States at (866) 744-2665, or outside the United States at (510) 253-0500.

Rockridge Press publishes its books in a variety of electronic and print formats. Some content that appears in print may not be available in electronic books, and vice versa.

Interior and Cover Designer: John Calmeyer
Art Producer: Sue Smith
Editor: Rachel Feldman
Production Manager: Oriana Siska
Production Editor: Erum Khan

Illustrations: © Paola Pardini/www.youworkforthem. com and © The Noun Project

ISBN: Print 978-1-64611-032-2

#dietGOALS

A Diet Journal for Your Weight Loss Journey

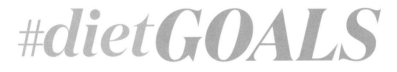

ROCKRIDGE
PRESS

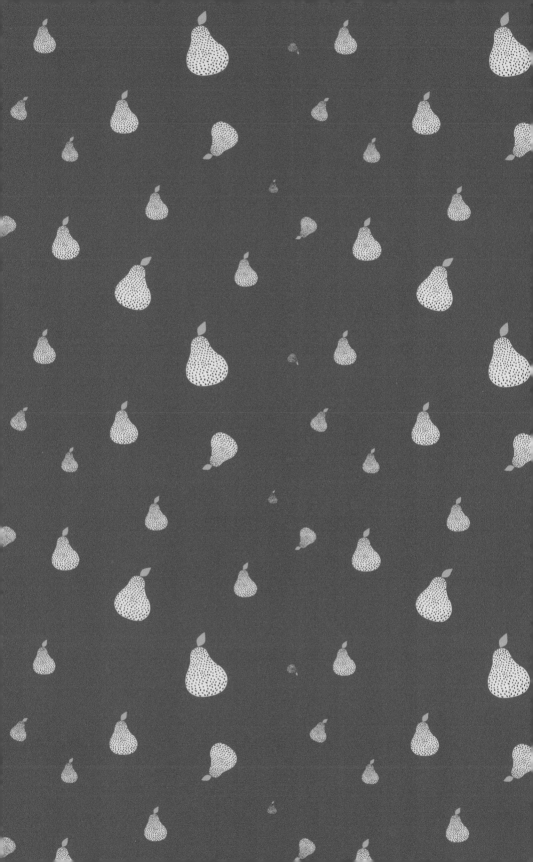

Starting Your Journey

If you're reading this, congratulations— you're already one step closer to your goal.

Whatever that goal may be—confidence, energy, overall health—this journal can be a powerful tool in helping you make it happen. At this point, you may still have doubts. How is a journal really going to help me? Why not just use a free app? Why track anything at all?

Here's why journaling is so powerful: This journal, which you will write in every single day for the next 12 weeks, represents a commitment to yourself. It's not easy to change your habits. Sometimes it can feel truly impossible. But recording and tracking the choices you make daily holds you accountable in a way that nothing else can. By designating a unique space that's solely for your important goal—without the distractions of other people or apps—you'll find yourself more committed than ever before.

As the days go by, you'll develop a new level of awareness. You'll be able to notice patterns and make positive changes. You'll stay motivated by seeing your progress week by week. But the most powerful thing this journal can do is give you the ability to look beyond numbers, beyond inches, beyond 90 days. To successfully change your life, you can't just meet your goal—you have to live within it. Journaling will help you commit to yourself daily so that you can do just that.

This journal is there for those moments when you feel like giving up, those moments when you're beaming with pride, and every single day in between. No matter where you're coming from, or what your goal is, this journal will be by your side during the journey. So go ahead and turn the page—it's time to write a new chapter in your life!

How to Use This Journal

Daily Entries

This journal is very intuitive to use, but here's a handy breakdown of a daily entry, as well as some tips for adapting it to your own journey:

1. Write down the date.

2. Record how many hours of sleep you got the night before.

3. Track how many glasses of water you drank.

4. Check off whether you took your daily meds or vitamins.

5. Log your breakfast, lunch, dinner, and snacks.

6. Include any optional information you want to track about your meals, like calories, macros, level of satisfaction, etc.

7. Record your daily activity.

8. Indicate your mood at the end of the day.

9. Reflect on the day in any way you want—explain your mood, set a goal for tomorrow, etc. If you had a particularly good or bad day, this is a helpful section where you can reflect on which factors played a role.

A Word about Diets...

No matter what your diet looks like, you can tailor this journal to your needs. You shouldn't feel the need to fill in every entry exactly as it's presented. If you're eating four bigger meals instead of three meals and snacks, you can use the snacks section to log your fourth meal. If you're intermittent fasting, feel free to skip the breakfast section and use that space for something else, like to log a mindful morning routine.

1 1/28 **2** 8 hrs. **3** ~~HHH~~ lll **4** ✓

Breakfast	Notes
coffee with half-and-half	25 cal
oatmeal with berries and almonds	270 cal

Lunch	
veggie buddha bowl with tofu	415 cal

5 **6**

Dinner	
baked salmon with sweet potatoes	410 cal
and broccoli	

Snacks	
1 cup of unsalted mixed nuts	160 cal
1 banana	105 cal
3 pieces of dark chocolate	170 cal

Activity

Ran 1 mile (12 minutes), then walked for another

20 minutes **7**

8 🤩 😊 😐 🙁 😭

Reflection

Ran out of energy on my run . . . try eating pre-run

snack closer to run time!

9

Setting Goals

How to Be S.M.A.R.T.

You may already be a goal-setting pro, but for those of you who are unsure of where to start, here's how to be S.M.A.R.T. The S.M.A.R.T. method, which has been around since the 1980s, involves using a specific set of criteria to achieve a goal:

Specific The more specific you are in setting your goal, the better the chance you have of attaining it.

Measurable What will your goal result in? By defining the results in very concrete ways, you'll be better able to identify how to get there, as well as refine exactly what it is you want to achieve.

Attainable Is your goal realistic and healthy? Does it take everything you're up against into account? It's never wrong to set a high goal, but if you set the bar too high, you'll only set yourself up for failure and get discouraged.

Relevant Why do you want to reach this goal? What is your ultimate objective? Will this goal really help with that? This is the part of your goal that keeps your "why" in check.

Timely This part is twofold. Yes, it's about making deadlines so that you'll feel motivated by a deeper sense of urgency. But it's also about not making your deadlines so tight that you'll get burnt out and give up.

Being S.M.A.R.T. is what making it happen is all about. By bringing structure and trackability to your goal, you'll be that much closer to making it real.

Weekly Challenges

This journal will suggest a healthy challenge for you every week, such as getting at least 20 minutes of activity in every day or trying a new healthy dish. But there's also space for you to add your own challenge or personal objective for the week.

My Goals

What is your overall goal?

....

....

....

What's the reason behind this goal, or your overall "why"?

....

....

....

Why are you starting this journey now?

....

....

....

What's your plan of action?

....

....

....

What are your biggest hurdles? What will help you along the way?

....

....

....

How will things be different?

....

....

....

15 Tips to Get Started

1 Start with small changes, one at a time, like eliminating sugary drinks or not eating after 9 p.m.

2 Tell yourself something positive right before you go to sleep and right when you wake up.

3 Set challenges or goals that make you excited, not anxious.

4 Plan your meals in advance as much as possible.

5 Spend 10 minutes stretching to some relaxing music in the morning.

6 Pack your meals with protein.

7 Stop looking at screens at least 30 minutes before you go to sleep. Try reading instead.

8 Put a quote or a photo that makes you happy in a place where you're always looking—the mirror, your phone or laptop background, etc.

9 Drink 8 glasses of water a day. Start getting into the habit by drinking a glass of water before every meal.

10 Try to understand your cravings. If you're craving chocolate all the time, you may need more magnesium in your diet. Try a handful of salty almonds instead.

11 Choose an activity that makes you happy, like dancing or gardening.

12 Find healthy foods that you love and indulge in them (a bowl of roasted veggies, etc.).

13 Practice eating slower. Enjoy every bite rather than rushing through a meal.

14 Start lifting weights. You'll feel powerful!

15 Make choices through positive reinforcement ("this makes me feel good") rather than negative reinforcement ("this is a punishment").

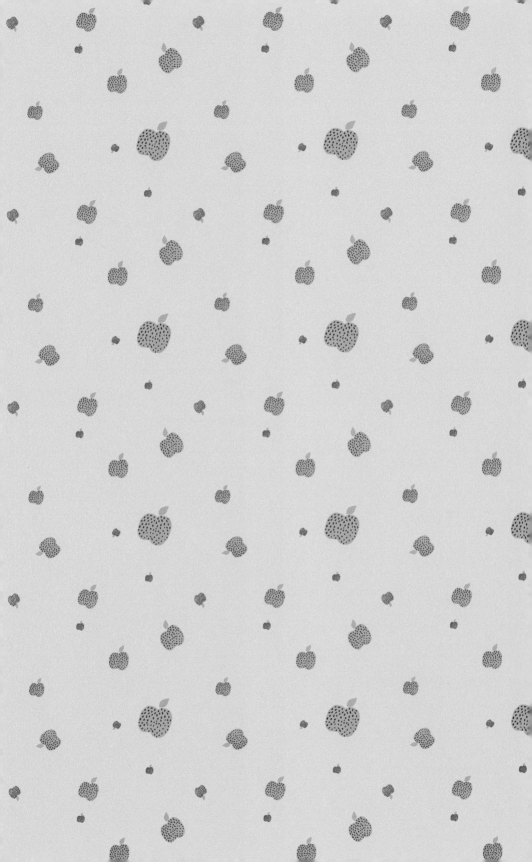

First Check-In

Date ....

Weight	
Upper Arms	
Chest	
Waist	
Hips	
Thighs	
Calves	

Describe how you feel about your current...

Stress levels

....

....

Confidence

....

....

Sleep schedule

....

....

Energy levels

....

....

Diet

....

....

Level of activity

....

....

How are you feeling overall right now?

....

....

First weekly challenge...

Write in your journal every day this week.

....

....

Ready to make it happen?

....

Breakfast

Notes

....

....

....

Lunch

....

....

....

Dinner

....

....

....

Snacks

....

....

....

Activity

....

....

....

Reflection

....

....

....

....

Breakfast   *Notes*

....
....
....

Lunch

....
....
....

Dinner

....
....
....

Snacks

....
....
....

Activity

....
....
....

Reflection

....
....
....

Motivation is what gets you started. Habit is what keeps you going.

—JIM RYUN

....

Breakfast

Notes

Lunch

Dinner

Snacks

Activity

Reflection

....

Breakfast

Notes

....

....

....

Lunch

....

....

....

Dinner

....

....

....

Snacks

....

....

....

Activity

....

....

....

Reflection

....

....

....

Breakfast	Notes

Lunch

Dinner

Snacks

Activity

Reflection

....

Breakfast   *Notes*
....
....
....

Lunch
....
....
....

Dinner
....
....
....

Snacks
....
....
....

Activity
....
....
....

Reflection
....
....
....

.... | .... | .... | ....

Breakfast

Notes

....

....

....

Lunch

....

....

....

Dinner

....

....

....

Snacks

....

....

....

Activity

....

....

....

Reflection

....

....

....

Weekly Check-In

Date .... Weight ....

Describe how you feel about your current...

Stress levels

....

....

....

Confidence

....

....

....

Sleep schedule

....

....

....

Energy levels

....

....

....

Diet

....

....

....

Level of activity

....

....

....

How did you feel about this week?

....

....

....

....

What were the highlights of the week?

....

....

....

....

What were the hardest parts of the week?

....

....

....

....

How do you feel about your overall goal?

....

....

....

....

Next weekly challenge...
Plan your weekly menu and shopping list.

....

....

....

Breakfast   *Notes*

....

....

....

Lunch

....

....

....

Dinner

....

....

....

Snacks

....

....

....

Activity

....

....

....

Reflection

....

....

....

....

Breakfast

Notes

....

....

....

Lunch

....

....

....

Dinner

....

....

....

Snacks

....

....

....

Activity

....

....

....

Reflection

....

....

....

There's no straighter road to success than exceeding expectations one day at a time.

—ROBIN CROW

....

Breakfast   *Notes*

....

....

....

Lunch

....

....

....

Dinner

....

....

....

Snacks

....

....

....

Activity

....

....

....

Reflection

....

....

....

....

Breakfast

Notes

....
....
....

Lunch

....
....
....

Dinner

....
....
....

Snacks

....
....
....

Activity

....
....
....

Reflection

....
....
....

....

Breakfast   Notes

....

....

....

Lunch

....

....

....

Dinner

....

....

....

Snacks

....

....

....

Activity

....

....

....

Reflection

....

....

....

....

Breakfast   **Notes**

....

....

....

Lunch

....

....

....

Dinner

....

....

....

Snacks

....

....

....

Activity

....

....

....

Reflection

....

....

....

....

Breakfast

Notes

....

....

....

Lunch

....

....

....

Dinner

....

....

....

Snacks

....

....

....

Activity

....

....

....

Reflection

....

....

....

Weekly Check-In

Date .... Weight ....

Describe how you feel about your current...

Stress levels

....

....

....

Confidence

....

....

....

Sleep schedule

....

....

....

Energy levels

....

....

....

Diet

....

....

....

Level of activity

....

....

....

How did you feel about this week?

....

....

....

....

What were the highlights of the week?

....

....

....

....

What were the hardest parts of the week?

....

....

....

....

How do you feel about your overall goal?

....

....

....

....

Next weekly challenge...
Try a new workout once this week.

....

....

....

Breakfast	*Notes*

Lunch	

Dinner	

Snacks	

Activity

Reflection

....

Breakfast

Notes

....

....

....

Lunch

....

....

....

Dinner

....

....

....

Snacks

....

....

....

Activity

....

....

....

Reflection

....

....

....

A goal without a plan is just a wish.

....

Breakfast

Notes

....

....

....

Lunch

....

....

....

Dinner

....

....

....

Snacks

....

....

....

Activity

....

....

....

Reflection

....

....

....

....

Breakfast	Notes

Lunch	

Dinner	

Snacks	

Activity

....

....

....

Reflection

....

....

....

....

Breakfast   *Notes*

....

....

....

Lunch

....

....

....

Dinner

....

....

....

Snacks

....

....

....

Activity

....

....

....

Reflection

....

....

....

....

Breakfast	Notes
....	....
....	....
....	....

Lunch

....	....
....	....
....	....

Dinner

....	....
....	....
....	....

Snacks

....	....
....	....
....	....

Activity

....
....
....

Reflection

....
....
....

....

Breakfast | Notes
....
....
....

Lunch
....
....
....

Dinner
....
....
....

Snacks
....
....
....

Activity
....
....
....

Reflection

....
....
....

Weekly Check-In

Date .... Weight ....

Describe how you feel about your current...

Stress levels

....
....
....

Confidence

....
....
....

Sleep schedule

....
....
....

Energy levels

....
....
....

Diet

....
....
....

Level of activity

....
....
....

How did you feel about this week?

....

....

....

What were the highlights of the week?

....

....

....

What were the hardest parts of the week?

....

....

....

How do you feel about your overall goal?

....

....

....

Next weekly challenge...

Be fully present at every meal—don't eat in bed or at your desk.

....

....

....

Breakfast   *Notes*

....

....

....

Lunch

....

....

....

Dinner

....

....

....

Snacks

....

....

....

Activity

....

....

....

Reflection

....

....

....

....

Breakfast	Notes
....	....
....	....
....	....

Lunch

.... | ....
.... | ....
.... | ....

Dinner

.... | ....
.... | ....
.... | ....

Snacks

.... | ....
.... | ....
.... | ....

Activity

....

....

....

Reflection

....

....

....

Strive for progress, not perfection.

Breakfast

Notes

Lunch

Dinner

Snacks

Activity

Reflection

....

Breakfast	Notes
....	....
....	....
....	....

Lunch	
....	....
....	....
....	....

Dinner	
....	....
....	....
....	....

Snacks	
....	....
....	....
....	....

Activity

....

....

....

Reflection

....

....

....

....

Breakfast

Notes

Lunch

Dinner

Snacks

Activity

Reflection

....

Breakfast   *Notes*

....

....

....

Lunch

....

....

....

Dinner

....

....

....

Snacks

....

....

....

Activity

....

....

....

Reflection

....

....

....

....

Breakfast   *Notes*

....

....

....

Lunch

....

....

....

Dinner

....

....

....

Snacks

....

....

....

Activity

....

....

....

Reflection

....

....

....

4-Week Check-In

Date ....

Weight	
Upper Arms	
Chest	
Waist	
Hips	
Thighs	
Calves	

How do you feel about the last four weeks?

....

....

....

What were the biggest challenges?

....

....

....

What are your proudest accomplishments?

....

....

....

How are you staying motivated?

....

....

....

What goals do you have for the next four weeks?

....

....

....

How do you feel about your overall goal?

....

....

....

How do you feel about your overall "why"?

....

....

....

Next weekly challenge...

Try a strength training routine.

....

....

*If you keep going
you won't regret it.
If you give up, you will.*

....

Breakfast

Notes

....

....

....

Lunch

....

....

....

Dinner

....

....

....

Snacks

....

....

....

Activity

....

....

....

Reflection

....

....

....

....

Breakfast   Notes

....

....

....

Lunch

....

....

....

Dinner

....

....

....

Snacks

....

....

....

Activity

....

....

....

Reflection

....

....

....

Discipline is greater than motivation.

....

Breakfast	Notes
....	....
....	....
....	....

Lunch

.... | ....
.... | ....
.... | ....

Dinner

.... | ....
.... | ....
.... | ....

Snacks

.... | ....
.... | ....
.... | ....

Activity

....
....
....

Reflection

....
....
....

Breakfast

Notes

Lunch

Dinner

Snacks

Activity

Reflection

Reflection

....

Breakfast

Notes

....

....

Lunch

....

....

....

Dinner

....

....

Snacks

....

....

....

Activity

....

....

....

Reflection

....

....

....

....

Breakfast   Notes

....

....

....

Lunch

....

....

....

Dinner

....

....

....

Snacks

....

....

....

Activity

....

....

....

Reflection

....

....

....

....

Breakfast

Notes

Lunch

Dinner

Snacks

Activity

Reflection

Weekly Check-In

Date .... Weight ....

Describe how you feel about your current...

Stress levels

....

....

....

Confidence

....

....

....

Sleep schedule

....

....

....

Energy levels

....

....

....

Diet

....

....

....

Level of activity

....

....

....

How did you feel about this week?

....

....

....

....

What were the highlights of the week?

....

....

....

....

What were the hardest parts of the week?

....

....

....

....

How do you feel about your overall goal?

....

....

....

....

Next weekly challenge...
Try cooking a new recipe.

....

....

....

Breakfast

Notes

....
....
....

Lunch

....
....
....

Dinner

....
....
....

Snacks

....
....
....

Activity

....
....
....

Reflection

....
....
....

....

Breakfast   *Notes*

Lunch

Dinner

Snacks

Activity

Reflection

*The past
is a place
of reference,
not a place
of residence.*

—ROY T. BENNETT

....

Breakfast

.... Notes

....

....

Lunch

....

....

....

Dinner

....

....

....

Snacks

....

....

....

Activity

....

....

....

Reflection

....

....

....

Breakfast   Notes

Lunch

Dinner

Snacks

Activity

Reflection

....

Breakfast   *Notes*

....
....
....

Lunch

....
....
....

Dinner

....
....
....

Snacks

....
....
....

Activity

....
....
....

Reflection

....
....
....

....

Breakfast   Notes

....

....

....

Lunch

....

....

....

Dinner

....

....

....

Snacks

....

....

....

Activity

....

....

....

Reflection

....

....

....

....

Breakfast

....

....

....

Lunch

....

....

....

Dinner

....

....

....

Snacks

....

....

....

Activity

....

....

....

Notes

....

....

....

Reflection

....

....

....

Weekly Check-In

Date .... Weight ....

Describe how you feel about your current...

Stress levels

....

....

....

Confidence

....

....

....

Sleep schedule

....

....

....

Energy levels

....

....

....

Diet

....

....

....

Level of activity

....

....

....

How did you feel about this week?

....

....

....

What were the highlights of the week?

....

....

....

What were the hardest parts of the week?

....

....

....

How do you feel about your overall goal?

....

....

....

Next weekly challenge...
Get at least 30 minutes of activity every single day this week.

....

....

....

Breakfast   Notes

....

....

....

Lunch

....

....

....

Dinner

....

....

....

Snacks

....

....

Activity

....

....

....

Reflection

....

....

....

....

Breakfast   *Notes*

....

....

....

Lunch

....

....

....

Dinner

....

....

....

Snacks

....

....

....

Activity

....

....

....

Reflection

....

....

....

Treating yourself means taking care of yourself.

....

Breakfast

Notes

....

....

....

Lunch

....

....

....

Dinner

....

....

....

Snacks

....

....

....

Activity

....

....

....

Reflection

....

....

....

....

Breakfast

Notes

....

....

....

Lunch

....

....

....

Dinner

....

....

....

Snacks

....

....

....

Activity

....

....

....

Reflection

....

....

....

....

Breakfast   *Notes*

....

....

....

Lunch

....

....

....

Dinner

....

....

....

Snacks

....

....

....

Activity

....

....

....

Reflection

....

....

....

....

Breakfast   Notes

....
....
....

Lunch

....
....
....

Dinner

....
....
....

Snacks

....
....
....

Activity

....
....
....

Reflection

....
....
....

....

Breakfast

Notes

Lunch

Dinner

Snacks

Activity

Reflection

Weekly Check-In

Date .... Weight ....

Describe how you feel about your current...

Stress levels

....

....

....

Confidence

....

....

....

Sleep schedule

....

....

....

Energy levels

....

....

....

Diet

....

....

....

Level of activity

....

....

....

How did you feel about this week?

....

....

....

....

What were the highlights of the week?

....

....

....

....

What were the hardest parts of the week?

....

....

....

....

How do you feel about your overall goal?

....

....

....

....

Next weekly challenge...
Eat protein-packed breakfasts every day this week.

....

....

....

Breakfast   **Notes**

....

....

....

Lunch

....

....

....

Dinner

....

....

....

Snacks

....

....

....

Activity

....

....

....

Reflection

....

....

....

....

Breakfast	Notes

Breakfast

.... | ....

.... | ....

.... | ....

Lunch

.... | ....

.... | ....

.... | ....

Dinner

.... | ....

.... | ....

.... | ....

Snacks

.... | ....

.... | ....

.... | ....

Activity

....

....

....

Reflection

....

....

....

You can't cross the sea merely by standing and staring at the water.

—RABINDRANATH TAGORE

....

Breakfast

Notes

....

....

....

Lunch

....

....

....

Dinner

....

....

....

Snacks

....

....

....

Activity

....

....

....

Reflection

....

....

....

....

Breakfast   Notes

....

....

Lunch

....

....

Dinner

....

....

Snacks

....

....

Activity

....

....

Reflection

....

....

....

....

Breakfast	Notes
....	....
....	....
....	....

Lunch

....	....
....	....
....	....

Dinner

....	....
....	....
....	....

Snacks

....	....
....	....
....	....

Activity

....

....

....

Reflection

....

....

....

....

Breakfast   *Notes*

....

....

....

Lunch

....

....

....

Dinner

....

....

....

Snacks

....

....

....

Activity

....

....

....

Reflection

....

....

....

....

Breakfast	Notes

....

....

....

Lunch

....

....

....

Dinner

....

....

....

Snacks

....

....

....

Activity

....

....

....

Reflection

....

....

....

4-Week Check-In

Date ....

Weight	
Upper Arms	
Chest	
Waist	
Hips	
Thighs	
Calves	

How do you feel about the last 4 weeks?

....

....

....

What were the biggest challenges?

....

....

....

What are your proudest accomplishments?

....

....

....

How are you staying motivated?

....

....

....

What goals do you have for the next four weeks?

....

....

....

How do you feel about your overall goal?

....

....

....

How do you feel about your overall "why"?

....

....

....

Next weekly challenge...

Drink a big glass of water as soon as you wake up every

morning next week.

....

*Remember where you
were eight weeks ago?
You're a different
person now. Own it!*

....

Breakfast   *Notes*

....

....

....

Lunch

....

....

....

Dinner

....

....

....

Snacks

....

....

....

Activity

....

....

....

Reflection

....

....

....

Breakfast   **Notes**

....
....
....

Lunch

....
....
....

Dinner

....
....
....

Snacks

....
....
....

Activity

....
....
....

Reflection

....
....
....

Loving ourselves works miracles in our lives.

—LOUISE HAY

....

Breakfast	Notes
....	....
....	....
....	....

Lunch	
....	....
....	....
....	....

Dinner	
....	....
....	....
....	....

Snacks	
....	....
....	....
....	....

Activity

....

....

....

Reflection

....

....

....

Breakfast   Notes

Lunch

Dinner

Snacks

Activity

Reflection

....

Breakfast   *Notes*

....

....

....

Lunch

....

....

....

Dinner

....

....

....

Snacks

....

....

....

Activity

....

....

....

Reflection

....

....

....

....

Breakfast   Notes

....

....

....

Lunch

....

....

....

Dinner

....

....

....

Snacks

....

....

....

Activity

....

....

....

Reflection

....

....

....

....

Breakfast   *Notes*

....

....

Lunch

....

....

Dinner

....

....

Snacks

....

....

Activity

....

....

....

Reflection

....

....

....

Weekly Check-In

Date .... Weight ....

Describe how you feel about your current...

Stress levels

....

....

Confidence

....

....

Sleep schedule

....

....

Energy levels

....

....

Diet

....

....

Level of activity

....

....

How did you feel about this week?

....

....

....

....

What were the highlights of the week?

....

....

....

....

What were the hardest parts of the week?

....

....

....

....

How do you feel about your overall goal?

....

....

....

....

Next weekly challenge...
Go to sleep 30 minutes earlier than you normally do every

night this week.

....

....

Breakfast   Notes

....

....

....

Lunch

....

....

....

Dinner

....

....

....

Snacks

....

....

....

Activity

....

....

....

Reflection

....

....

....

....

Breakfast

Notes

Lunch

Dinner

Snacks

Activity

Reflection

It's not about having enough time, it's about making enough time.

—RACHAEL BERMINGHAM

....

Breakfast | Notes

Lunch

Dinner

Snacks

Activity

Reflection

Breakfast

Notes

Lunch

Dinner

Snacks

Activity

Reflection

....

Breakfast

....

....

....

Lunch

....

....

....

Dinner

....

....

....

Snacks

....

....

....

Activity

....

....

....

Notes

Reflection

....

....

....

....

Breakfast   *Notes*

....

....

....

Lunch

....

....

....

Dinner

....

....

....

Snacks

....

....

....

Activity

....

....

....

Reflection

....

....

....

....

Breakfast   *Notes*

....

....

....

Lunch

....

....

....

Dinner

....

....

....

Snacks

....

....

....

Activity

....

....

....

Reflection

....

....

....

Weekly Check-In

Date .... Weight ....

Describe how you feel about your current...

Stress levels

....

....

....

Confidence

....

....

....

Sleep schedule

....

....

....

Energy levels

....

....

....

Diet

....

....

....

Level of activity

....

....

....

How did you feel about this week?

....

....

....

What were the highlights of the week?

....

....

....

What were the hardest parts of the week?

....

....

....

How do you feel about your overall goal?

....

....

....

....

Next weekly challenge...
Plan "me" time this week—take a bath, go on a long walk,

get a massage, see a movie, or do some people watching at a café.

....

....

Breakfast   *Notes*

....
....
....

Lunch

....
....
....

Dinner

....
....
....

Snacks

....
....
....

Activity

....
....
....

Reflection

....
....
....

....

Breakfast   Notes

....

....

....

Lunch

....

....

....

Dinner

....

....

....

Snacks

....

....

....

Activity

....

....

....

Reflection

....

....

....

Don't compare yourself to others. Compare yourself to the person from yesterday.

....

Breakfast	Notes
....	....
....	....
....	....

Lunch	
....	....
....	....
....	....

Dinner	
....	....
....	....
....	....

Snacks	
....	....
....	....
....	....

Activity

....

....

....

Reflection

....

....

....

....

Breakfast   *Notes*

....
....
....

Lunch

....
....
....

Dinner

....
....
....

Snacks

....
....
....

Activity

....
....
....

Reflection

....
....
....

Breakfast

Notes

Lunch

Dinner

Snacks

Activity

Reflection

Reflection

.... | .... | .... | ....

Breakfast

Notes

....
....
....

Lunch

....
....
....

Dinner

....
....
....

Snacks

....
....
....

Activity

....
....
....

Reflection

....
....
....

....

Breakfast   *Notes*

....

....

....

Lunch

....

....

....

Dinner

....

....

....

Snacks

....

....

....

Activity

....

....

....

Reflection

....

....

....

Weekly Check-In

Date .... Weight ....

Describe how you feel about your current...

Stress levels

....

....

....

Confidence

....

....

....

Sleep schedule

....

....

....

Energy levels

....

....

....

Diet

....

....

....

Level of activity

....

....

....

How did you feel about this week?

....

....

....

....

What were the highlights of the week?

....

....

....

....

What were the hardest parts of the week?

....

....

....

....

How do you feel about your overall goal?

....

....

....

....

Next weekly challenge...
Try eating only whole foods this week (nothing in a package).

....

....

....

Breakfast	Notes
....	....
....	....

Lunch	
....	....
....	....

Dinner	
....	....
....	....

Snacks	
....	....
....	....

Activity

....

....

Reflection

....

....

....

....

Breakfast   *Notes*

....
....
....

Lunch

....
....
....

Dinner

....
....
....

Snacks

....
....
....

Activity

....
....
....

Reflection

....
....
....

The moment when you want to quit is the moment when you need to keep pushing.

....

Breakfast   Notes

....

....

....

Lunch

....

....

....

Dinner

....

....

....

Snacks

....

....

....

Activity

....

....

....

Reflection

....

....

....

....

Breakfast   *Notes*

....

....

....

Lunch

....

....

....

Dinner

....

....

....

Snacks

....

....

....

Activity

....

....

....

Reflection

....

....

....

....

Breakfast	Notes
....	....
....	....
	....

Lunch	
....	....
....	....
	....

Dinner	
....	....
....	....
	....

Snacks	
....	....
....	....
	....

Activity

....

....

....

Reflection

....

....

....

....

Breakfast *Notes*

....

....

....

Lunch

....

....

....

Dinner

....

....

....

Snacks

....

....

....

Activity

....

....

....

Reflection

....

....

....

Breakfast

Notes

Lunch

Dinner

Snacks

Activity

Reflection

Final Check-In

Date ....

Weight	
Upper Arms	
Chest	
Waist	
Hips	
Thighs	
Calves	

How do you feel about the last 12 weeks?

....

....

....

What were the biggest challenges?

....

....

....

What are your proudest accomplishments?

....

....

....

How do you feel about your goal?

....

....

....

How do you feel about your "why"?

....

....

....

What's next?

....

....

....

You made it happen.
Don't stop here—go live your goal!

References

AZ Quotes. "Robin Crow Quote." Accessed 2019. https://www.azquotes.com/quote/881307.

Goodreads. "Quotes by Rachael Bermingham." Accessed 2019. www.goodreads.com/quotes/609982-it-s-not-about-having-enough-time-it-s-about-making-enough.

Goodreads. "Quote By Roy T. Bennett." Accessed 2019. https://www.goodreads.com/quotes/7987120-the-past-is-a-place-of-reference-not-a-place.

Kaiser, Shannon. "12 Quotes From Louise Hay That Will Inspire You To Love Yourself Right Now." Huffpost. September 9, 2017. https://www.huffpost.com/entry/12-quotes-from-louise-hay-that-will-inspire-you-to_b_59b44533e4b0c50640cd67d7.

Wei, Jessica. "Motivation Is What Gets You Started—Jim Ryun," *Due* (blog), January 16, 2016. https://due.com/blog/motivation-gets-started-jim-ryun.

"Words of Wisdom: Rabindranath Tagore's Famous and Inspirational Quotes," *India Today*, August 6, 2016. https://www.indiatoday.in/education-today/gk-current-affairs/story/tagore-quotes-333701-2016-08-06.